Anti-Inflammatory Diet

How To Defeat The Symptoms Of Inflammation And Your
Hypertension By Restoring Your Health Step By Step

(The Comprehensive Guide On Anti Inflammatory Diet)

Ricky Hughes

Table Of Contents

Barley Porridge

Ingredients:

- 2 cups of water
- Toppings such as hazelnuts, honey, berry, etc.
- 1 cup barley
- 1 cup of wheat berries
- 2 cups unsweetened almond milk

Directions:

1. Take a medium saucepan and place it over medium-high heat
2. Place barley, almond milk, wheat berries, water and bring to a boil
3. Lower down the heat to low and simmer for 25 minutes

4. Divide amongst serving bowls and top with your desired toppings. Serve and enjoy!

Hearty Fresh Banana Oatmeal

Ingredients:

- 2 tablespoon of flaxseeds, ground
- 2 tablespoon of chia seeds
- 2 bananas, peeled and mashed
- 1 teaspoon of vanilla extract
- 1 teaspoon of cinnamon powder
- 2 cups of water
- 1 cup steel-cut oats 1 cup of almond milk
- 1/2 cup walnuts, chopped

Directions:

1. Add water, oats, almond milk, flaxseed, walnuts, chia seeds, vanilla,

bananas, cinnamon to your Pot and give it a nice toss Lock up the lid and cook on HIGH pressure for 10 minutes Release the pressure naturally and open the lid Divide the mix amongst bowls and serve Enjoy!

Pumpkin And Cinnamon Porridge Meal

Ingredients:

1 teaspoon ground cinnamon

2 tablespoon ground flaxseed meal

Juice of 1 lemon

1 cup pumpkin puree

1 cup unsweetened almond/coconut milk

1 cup of water 1 cup uncooked quinoa

Directions:

2. Take a pot and place it over medium-high heat
3. Whisk in water, almond milk and bring the mix to a boil
4. Stir in quinoa, cinnamon, and pumpkin
5. Lower heat to low and simmer for 10 minutes until the liquid has been evaporated
6. Remove heat and stir in flaxseed meal
7. Transfer porridge to small bowls
8. Sprinkle lemon juice and add pumpkin seeds on top.
9. Serve and enjoy!

Scrambled Turkey Eggs

Ingredients:

1 medium yellow onion, diced

1/2 teaspoon hot pepper sauce

3 large free-range eggs 1/2 teaspoon salt

1/2 teaspoon black pepper, freshly ground

1 tablespoon coconut oil

1 medium red bell pepper, diced

Directions:

1. Set a pan to medium-high heat and add coconut oil, let it heat up
2. Add onions and Sauté
3. Add turkey and red pepper
4. Cook until turkey is cooked

5. Take a bowl and beat eggs, stir in salt and pepper
6. Pour eggs in the pan with turkey and gently cook and scramble eggs
7. Top with hot sauce and enjoy!

Cinnamon Baked Apple Chips

Ingredients:

2 2 apples

1 teaspoon cinnamon

Directions:

1. Preheat your oven to 200 degrees Fahrenheit
2. Take a sharp knife and slice apples into thin slices
3. Discard seeds
4. Line a baking sheet with parchment paper and arrange apples on it
5. Make sure they do not overlap
6. Once done, sprinkle cinnamon over apples
7. Bake in the oven for 1 hour

8. Flip and bake for an hour more until no longer moist
9. Serve and enjoy!

Herb And Avocado Omelet

Ingredients:

1 cup almonds, sliced

Salt and pepper as needed

3 large free-range eggs

1 medium avocado, sliced

Directions:

1. Take a non-stick skillet and place it over medium-high heat
2. Take a bowl and add eggs, beat the eggs

3. Pour to the skillet and cook for 1 minute
4. Lower heat to low and cook for 4 minutes
5. Top the omelet with almonds and avocado
6. Sprinkle salt and pepper and serve
7. Enjoy!

The Blueberry And Avocado Medley

Ingredients:

2 cups berries

Maple syrup as needed

1 frozen fresh Banana

2 avocados, quartered

Directions:

1. Take your blender and add all Ingredients except maple syrup
2. Add ice water and blend
3. Garnish with syrup and pour in smoothie glasses

Lovely Pumpkin Oats

Ingredients:

1 cup canned pumpkin puree

1/2 teaspoon pumpkin pie spice

1 teaspoon ground cinnamon

1 cup quick-cooking rolled oats

¾ cup almond milk

Directions:

1. Take a safe microwave bowl and add oats, almond milk, and microwave on high for 2 2 minutes
2. Add more almond milk if needed to achieve your desired consistency
3. Cook for 30 seconds more
4. Stir in pumpkin puree, pumpkin pie spice, ground cinnamon
5. Heat gently and enjoy!

Cool Cinnamon And Pear Oatmeal

Ingredients:

1 tablespoon cinnamon powder

1 cup pear, cored and peeled, cubed

3 cups of water

1 cup steel-cut oats

Directions:

1. Take a pot and add water, oats, cinnamon, pear and toss well
2. Bring it to simmer over medium heat
3. Let it cook for 15 minutes, divide amongst the bowl

Healthy Zucchini Stir Fry

Ingredients:

- 1 whole tablespoon of coconut aminos
- 1 whole tablespoon of a sesame seed, toasted
- Ground pepper (black) as much as needed
- 2 tablespoons of heaping olive oil
- 1 whole medium-sized onion, sliced thinly
- 2 whole medium-sized zucchini, cut up into thin sized strips
- 2 heaping tablespoons of teriyaki flavored sauce, low sodium

Directions:

1. Take a skillet and place it over medium level heat.
2. Add onions, and stir cook for 5 minutes
3. Add your zucchini and stir cook for 1 minute more.
4. Gently add the sauces alongside the sesame seeds
5. Cook for 5 minutes more until the zucchini are soft
6. Finally, add in pepper and enjoy!

Simple Blueberry Oatmeal

Ingredients:

1 cup of coconut milk

2 tablespoons agave nectar

1 teaspoon vanilla extract

Coconut flakes, garnish

1 cup blueberries

1 cup steel-cut oats

Directions:

1. Grease Slow Cooker with cooking spray
2. Add oats, milk, nectar, blueberries, and vanilla
3. Toss well
4. Place lid and cook on LOW for 8 hours

5. Divide between serving bowls and serve

Smoothie Bowl

Ingredients:

2 tablespoons flaxseed oil

2 tablespoons chia seeds

2 tablespoons walnuts, roughly chopped

A handful of fresh berries

2 cups baby spinach leaves

1 cup coconut almond milk

1/2 cup low fat cream

Directions:

1. Add spinach leaves, coconut almond milk, cream and flaxseed oil to a blender
2. Blitz until smooth
3. Pour smoothie into serving bowls
4. Sprinkle chia seeds, berries, walnuts on top
5. Serve and enjoy!

Salmon And Sweet Potato Mix

Ingredients:

1 tablespoon chopped chives

2 teaspoons horseradish

1/2 cup coconut cream

Salt and black pepper to the taste

1 tablespoon olive oil

11 pounds sweet potatoes, baked and cubed

4 ounces smoked salmon, chopped

Directions:

1. In a bowl, whisk together the coconut cream with salt, pepper, horseradish and chives.
2. Add salmon and potatoes, toss to coat and serve right away. Enjoy!

Cod And Tarragon Sauce

Ingredients:

- 4 tablespoons olive oil+ 1 teaspoon
- Salt and black pepper to the taste
- 2 cups lettuce leaves, torn
- 1 small red onion, sliced
- 1 small cucumber, sliced
- 2 tablespoons lemon juice 2 tablespoons water
- 2 tablespoons mustard
- 4 medium cod fillets, skinless and boneless
- 1 tablespoon chopped tarragon
- 1 tablespoon capers, drained

Directions:

1. In a bowl, mix mustard with 2 tablespoons olive oil, tarragon, capers and water, whisk well and set aside.
2. Heat up a pan with 1 teaspoon oil over medium-high heat.
3. Season fish with salt and pepper to the taste then add to pan and cook for 6 minutes on each side.
4. In a separate bowl, mix cucumber with onion, lettuce, lemon juice, 2 tablespoons olive oil, salt and pepper to the taste.
5. Arrange the cod between plates, drizzle the tarragon sauce all over and serve with the cucumber salad on the side. Enjoy!

Shrimp And Mango Mix

Ingredients:

4 cucumbers, peeled and cubed

1 mango, peeled and cubed

3 tablespoons chopped dill

2 pound shrimp, cooked, peeled and deveined

A pinch of salt and black pepper

2 tablespoons Dijon mustard

3 tablespoons white wine vinegar

6 tablespoons avocado mayonnaise

Directions:

1. In a salad bowl, mix the cucumbers with the mango, shrimp, dill, salt and pepper and toss. Add the mustard,

23

vinegar and mayonnaise and mix well then serve.

Orange Chicken Salad

Ingredients:

1/2 cup avocado mayonnaise

1 cup coconut cream

1 cup chopped cashews, toasted

A pinch of salt and black pepper

1 whole chicken, cut into medium pieces

4 scallions, chopped

2 celery ribs, chopped

1 cup chopped mandarin orange

Directions:

1. Put chicken pieces in a pot and add water to cover.
2. Add a pinch of salt then bring to a boil over medium heat and cook for 25 minutes.
3. Transfer to a cutting board, discard bones, shred meat and put in a bowl.
4. Add celery, orange pieces, cashews, scallion, salt, pepper, mayo and the coconut cream, toss to coat and serve.

Brown Rice And Chicken Mix

Ingredients:

2 tablespoon coconut aminos

4 ounces chicken breast boneless, skinless and cut into small pieces

1 fresh egg

2 fresh egg whites

2 scallions, chopped

11 cups brown rice, cooked

11 tablespoons coconut sugar

1 cup chicken stock

Directions:

1. Put stock in a pot, heat up over medium-low heat and add coconut aminos and sugar, stir, bring to a boil, add the chicken and toss. In a bowl, mix the fresh egg with fresh egg whites, whisk well then add over the chicken mix.
2. Sprinkle the scallions on top and cook for 3 minutes without stirring.
3. Divide the rice into 4 bowls, add the chicken mix on top and serve.

Greek Chicken Breasts

Ingredients:

2 teaspoons chopped thyme

1 cup chopped yellow fresh onion

3 garlic cloves, minced

1 cup kalamata olives, pitted and sliced

1/2 cup chopped parsley

3 cups chopped tomatoes

6 chicken breast halves, skinless and boneless

2 teaspoons olive oil

1 cup vegetable stock

1 tablespoon chopped basil

Directions:

1. Heat up a pan with the oil over medium heat, add chicken and cook for 6 minutes on each side.
2. Transfer cooked chicken to a plate. Heat up the same pan used for the chicken over medium heat, add garlic, stir and cook for 1 minute.
3. Add onion, tomatoes and the stock then stir and bring to a simmer.
4. Cook for 10 minutes.

5. Add basil, thyme and the chicken, mix and cook for 12 minutes.
6. Add parsley, olives, salt and pepper, toss, divide between plates and serve.

Enjoy!

Easy Chicken And Potato Mix

Ingredients:

2 pounds chicken breast, skinless, boneless and cubed

1 cup sliced red fresh onion

¾ cup vegetable stock

1 cup pepperoncini peppers, chopped

2 cups chopped tomato

1/2 cup kalamata olives, pitted and halved

2 tablespoons chopped basil

14 ounces canned artichokes, drained and chopped

1 tablespoon olive oil

4 teaspoons garlic, minced

A pinch of salt and black pepper

1/2 teaspoon dried thyme

12 small red potatoes, halved

Cooking spray

Directions:

1. In a baking dish, mix potatoes with 2 teaspoons garlic, olive oil, thyme, salt and pepper. Bake in the oven at 450 degrees F for 30 minutes.

2. Heat up a pot over medium-high heat, grease with cooking spray, add chicken, season with salt and black pepper and cook for 5 minutes on each side then transfer to a plate.
3. Heat up the pot again over medium heat, add onion, stir and cook for 5 minutes.
4. Add stock and return the chicken to the pot.
5. Add olives, pepperoncini and roasted potatoes, stir and cook for 3 minutes. Add the rest of the garlic, artichokes, basil and the tomatoes, stir, cook for 3 minutes. Divide between plates and serve.

Paprika Chicken Mix

Ingredients:

1 tablespoon olive oil

1 and 1 cups chicken stock

4 chicken breasts, skinless and boneless

1/2 teaspoon sweet paprika

1/3 cup mustard

Salt and black pepper to the taste

1 cup yellow onion, chopped

Directions:

1. In a bowl, whisk the paprika with mustard, salt and pepper.
2. Spread the mix over the chicken and rub well. Heat up a pan with the oil over medium-high heat, add chicken

breasts and cook for 2 minutes on each side then transfer to a plate. Heat up the pan once again over medium-high heat, add stock, stir and bring to a simmer.

3. Add onions, salt, pepper and return the chicken to the pan as well. Stir the mix and bring to a simmer over medium heat for 25 minutes, turning meat halfway.

4. Divide between plates, drizzle the sauce over it and serve.

Veggie Lunch Salad

Ingredients:

1/2 teaspoon matcha powder
1 teaspoon maple syrup
2 tablespoons white wine vinegar
1 tablespoon Dijon mustard
1/2 cup lemon juice   ¾ cup olive oil
2 carrots, peeled and grated

1 avocado, pitted, peeled and chopped

1 green cabbage head, shredded

10 strawberries, halved
Salt and black pepper to the taste

Directions:

1. In a bowl, whisk together the lemon juice with oil, vinegar, matcha tea powder, maple syrup, mustard, salt

and pepper. In a salad bowl, mix avocado with cabbage, strawberries and carrots.

2. Add lemon juice, oil, vinegar, matcha powder, maple syrup, mustard, salt and pepper. Toss well and serve for lunch. Enjoy!

Grilled Eggplant Lunch Salad

Ingredients:

1 teaspoon chopped oregano

3 tablespoons olive oil

2 garlic cloves, minced

3 tablespoons chopped parsley

2 tablespoons chopped capers

1 tomato, diced

1 eggplant, pricked

A pinch of salt and black pepper

1/2 teaspoon ground turmeric

11 teaspoons red wine vinegar

Directions:

1. Heat up your grill over medium-high heat, add eggplant, cook for 15 minutes, turning from time to time, scoop flesh, roughly chop and put in a bowl.
2. Add salt, pepper to the taste, tomatoes, turmeric, garlic, vinegar, oregano, parsley, oil and capers, toss and serve.

Eggplant And Avocado Lunch Mix

Ingredients:

1 tablespoon chopped oregano

1 teaspoon raw honey

A pinch of salt and black pepper

1 tablespoon chopped parsley

Zest of 1 lemon

1 eggplant, sliced

1 red onion, sliced

2 teaspoons olive oil

1 avocado, pitted and chopped

1 teaspoon mustard

1 tablespoon red wine vinegar

Directions:

1. Brush the fresh onion slices and eggplant slices with the olive oil, place them on the preheated kitchen grill, cook for 5 minutes on each side and let cool down.
2. Cut the veggies into cubes, put in a salad bowl, add avocado and toss. In a bowl, mix vinegar with mustard, oregano, honey, olive oil, salt and

pepper, whisk well and add to the salad.
3. Toss together and sprinkle the lemon zest and the parsley on top and serve.

Enjoy!

Eggplant And Fresh Egg Mix

Ingredients:

1/3 cup pine nuts   1/2 cup mustard

1 cup chopped sun-dried tomatoes

1 cup halved walnuts   1/2 cup olive oil

1 big purple eggplant, cubed

12 eggs, hard-boiled, peeled and cubed

Juice of 1 lemon

A pinch of salt and white pepper

Directions:

1. Spread eggplant cubes on a lined baking sheet.
2. In a bowl, whisk together half of the lemon juice with the oil, salt and pepper.
3. Pour the mix over the eggplant cubes, toss to coat, introduce in the oven at 450 degrees F and bake for 30 minutes.
4. In a food processor, mix the rest of the lemon juice, mustard, salt, pepper, walnuts, tomatoes and pine nuts and pulse well.
5. Put the eggs in a bowl, add eggplant cubes, mustard mix, toss to coat well and serve. Enjoy!

Stuffed Eggplants

Ingredients:

1 tablespoon lemon juice

1/2 teaspoon sweet paprika

1/2 teaspoon ground turmeric

A pinch of salt and black pepper

2 tablespoons olive oil

6 baby eggplants, halved

2 garlic cloves, minced

1 pound ground turkey

1 tablespoon chopped oregano

Directions:

1. Heat up a pan with the oil over medium heat, add the ground turkey, stir and cook for 5-6 minutes.

2. Add the oregano, lemon juice, paprika, turmeric, salt and pepper, stir, and cook for 5-6 minutes more.
3. Take off the heat, cool the mix down and stuff the eggplants with this mix.
4. Arrange the stuffed eggplants on a lined baking sheet, bake in the oven at 450 degrees F for 30 minutes then divide between plates and serve.

Veggie Soup

Ingredients:

A pinch of salt and black pepper

4 garlic cloves, minced

4 ounces kale, chopped

1 cup canned tomatoes, chopped

1 zucchini, chopped 2 quart veggie stock

A handful parsley, chopped for serving

1 yellow onion, chopped

2 carrots, chopped 6 mushrooms, chopped

1 red chili pepper, chopped

2 celery sticks, chopped

1 tablespoon coconut oil

Directions:

1. Heat up a pot with the oil over medium-high heat, add the celery, carrots, onion, salt and black pepper. Stir and cook for 2 minutes.
2. Add chili pepper, garlic, and mushrooms, stir and cook for 2 minutes.
3. Add tomatoes, stock, kale and zucchinis, stir then bring to a simmer.
4. Cook for 25 minutes, divide into bowls, sprinkle the parsley on top and serve.

Shrimp Soup

Ingredients:

2 cups chicken stock

Juice of 1 lime 15 cups coconut milk

2 pound shrimp, peeled and deveined

1 cup coconut cream

1 broccoli head, florets separated

1 zucchini, chopped 1 carrot, chopped

1 tablespoon parsley, chopped

5 tablespoons curry paste

1 tablespoon coconut oil

1 big chicken breast, cut into thin strips

4 tablespoons coconut aminos

Directions:

1. Heat up a pot with the oil over medium heat, add curry paste, stir and cook for 1 minute.
2. Add chicken, stock and lime juice. Stir and cook for 2 minutes.
3. Add coconut cream, aminos and coconut milk, stir and cook for 10 minutes.
4. Add broccoli florets, carrots, shrimp and zucchini, stir and cook for 4 minutes.
5. Ladle into bowls, top with parsley and serve. Enjoy!

46.   Chicken And Veggies

Ingredients:

1 tsp. Italian seasoning

14 oz. chopped no-salt-added canned tomatoes

4 de-boned, skinless and cubed chicken breasts

1/2 tsp. black pepper

1 c. chopped yellow fresh onion

16 oz. cauliflower florets

2 tbsps. Organic olive oil

Directions:

1. Heat up a pan while using the oil over medium-high heat, add chicken, black

pepper, fresh onion and Italian seasoning, toss and cook for 5 minutes.

2. Add tomatoes and cauliflower, toss, cover the pan and cook over medium heat for twenty possibly even minutes.

3. Toss again, divide everything between plates and serve.

Hidden Valley Chicken Drummies

Ingredients:

2 packages Hidden Valley dressing dry mix

3 tbsps. Vinegar

12 chicken drumsticks

Paprika

2 tbsps. Hot sauce

1 c. melted butter

Celery sticks

50

Directions:

1. Preheat the oven to 350 0F.
2. Rinse and pat dry the chicken.
3. In a bowl blend the dry dressing, melted butter, vinegar and hot sauce. Stir until combined.
4. Place the drumsticks in a large plastic baggie, pour the sauce over drumsticks. Massage the sauce until the drumsticks are coated.
5. Place the chicken in a single layer on a baking dish. Sprinkle with paprika.
6. Bake for 30 minutes, flipping halfway.
7. Serve with crudité or salad.

Lemon-Parsley Chicken Breast

Ingredients:

3 tbsps. Bread crumbs

2 skinless and boneless chicken breasts

2 minced garlic cloves

2 tbsps. Flavorless oil

1/3 c. lemon juice

1/2 c. fresh parsley

1/3 c. white wine

Directions:

1. Combine the wine, lemon juice and garlic in a measuring cup.
2. Pound each chicken breast, until they are 1/2 inch thick.

3. Coat the chicken with bread crumbs, and heat the oil in a large skillet.
4. Fry the chicken for 6 minutes on each side, until they turn brown.
5. Stir in the wine mixture over the chicken.
6. Simmer for 5 minutes
7. Serve. Pour any extra juices over the chicken. Garnish with parsley.

Lemony Mussels

Ingredients:

2 lbs. scrubbed mussels

Juice of one lemon

1 tbsp. extra virgin extra virgin olive oil

2 minced garlic cloves

Directions:

1. Put some water in a pot, add mussels, bring with a boil over medium heat, cook for 5 minutes, discard unopened mussels and transfer them with a bowl.
2. In another bowl, mix the oil with garlic and freshly squeezed lemon juice, whisk well, and add over the mussels, toss and serve.

Hot Tuna Steak

Ingredients:

1/2 c. whole black peppercorns

6 sliced tuna steaks

2 tbsps. Extra-virgin olive oil

Salt

2 tbsps. Fresh lemon juice

Pepper. Roasted orange garlic mayonnaise

Directions:

1. Place the tuna in a bowl to fit.
2. Add the oil, lemon juice, salt and pepper.
3. Turn the tuna to coat well in the marinade.
4. Let rest 25 to 30 minutes, turning once. Place the peppercorns in a double thickness of plastic bags.
5. Tap the peppercorns with a heavy saucepan or small mallet to crush them coarsely.
6. Place on a large plate. When ready to cook the tuna, dip the edges into the crushed peppercorns.

7. Heat a nonstick skillet over medium heat.
8. Sear the tuna steaks, in batches if necessary, for 4 minutes per side for medium-rare fish, adding 2 to 3 tablespoons of the marinade to the skillet if necessary, to prevent sticking. Serve dolloped with roasted orange garlic mayonnaise

Marinated Fish Steaks

Ingredients:

1 tbsp. snipped fresh oregano

1 lb. fresh swordfish

1 tsp. lemon-pepper seasoning

4 lime wedges

2 tbsps. Lime juice

2 minced garlic cloves 2 tsps. Olive oil

Directions:

1. Rinse fish steaks; pat dry wi th paper towels.
2. Cut into four serving size pieces, if necessary.
3. In a shallow dish combine lime juice, oregano, oil, lemon-pepper seasoning, and garlic.

4. Add fish; turn to coat with marinade. Cover and marinate in refrigerator for 30 minutes to 2 1/2 hours, turning steaks occasionally.
5. Drain fish, reserving marinade. Place fish on the greased unheated rack of a broiler pan.
6. Broil 4 inches from the heat for 8 to 12 minutes or until fish begins to flake when tested with a fork, turning once and brushing with reserved marinade halfway through cooking.
7. Discard any remaining marinade. Before serving, squeeze the juice from one lime wedge over each steak.

Lime Pork And Green Beans

Ingredients:

2 tablespoons lime juice

1 cup coconut milk

1 tablespoon rosemary, chopped

A pinch of salt and black pepper

2 pounds pork stew meat, cubed

2 tablespoons avocado oil

1 cup green beans, trimmed and halved

Directions:

1. Heat up a pan with the oil over medium heat, add the meat and brown for 5 minutes.

2. Add the rest of the ingredients, toss gently, bring to a simmer and cook over medium heat for 35 minutes more.
3. Divide the mix between plates and serve.

Pork With Lemongrass

Ingredients:

1 cup vegetable stock

1 stalk lemongrass, chopped

2 tablespoons coconut aminos

2 tablespoons cilantro, chopped

4 pork chops

2 tablespoons olive oil

2 spring onions, chopped

A pinch of salt and black pepper

Directions:

1. Heat up a pan with the oil over medium-high heat, add the spring onions and the meat and brown for 5 minutes.
2. Add the rest of the ingredients, toss, and cook everything over medium heat for 25 minutes more.
3. Divide the mix between plates and serve.

Pork With Olives

Ingredients:

1 tablespoon sweet paprika

2 tablespoons balsamic vinegar

1/2 cup kalamata olives, pitted and chopped

1 tablespoon cilantro, chopped

A pinch of sea salt and black pepper

1 yellow onion, chopped

4 pork chops

2 tablespoons olive oil

Directions:

1. Heat up a pan with the oil over medium heat, add the fresh onion and sauté for 5 minutes.
2. Add the meat and brown for 5 minutes more.
3. Add the rest of the ingredients, toss, cook over medium heat for 30 minutes, divide between plates and serve.

Pork Chops With Tomato Salsa

Ingredients:

A pinch of sea salt and black pepper

1 small red onion, chopped

2 tomatoes, cubed 2 tablespoons lime juice

1 jalapeno, chopped

1/2 cup cilantro, chopped

1 tablespoon lime juice

4 pork chops

1 tablespoon olive oil 4 scallions, chopped

1 teaspoon cumin, ground

1 tablespoon hot paprika

1 teaspoon garlic powder

65

Directions:

1. Heat up a pan with the oil over medium heat, add the scallions and sauté for 5 minutes.
2. Add the meat, cumin paprika, garlic powder, salt and pepper, toss, cook for 5 minutes on each side and divide between plates.
3. In a bowl, combine the tomatoes with the remaining ingredients, toss, divide next to the pork chops and serve.

Cabbage Orange Salad With Citrusy Vinaigrette

Ingredients:

1 teaspoon raspberry vinegar

2 tablespoons of fresh orange juice

2 oranges, peeled, sliced into pieces

1 tablespoon of honey

1/4 teaspoon of salt

Freshly ground pepper

4 teaspoons of olive oil

1 teaspoon orange zest,grated

2 tablespoons vegetable stock,reduced-sodium

1 teaspoon each cider vinegar

4 cups red cabbage, shredded

1 teaspoon lemon juice

1 fennel bulb, sliced thinly

1 teaspoon balsamic vinegar

Directions:

1. Put the following in a bowl and whisk – lemon juice, orange zest, cider vinegar, salt and pepper, broth, oil, honey, orange juice, balsamic vinegar and raspberry vinegar.
2. Extract the oranges, fennel and cabbage. Toss to coat.

Lemon Buttery Shrimp Rice

Ingredients:

1/2 cup frozen peas, thawed, rinsed, drained

1 Tbsp. lemon juice, freshly squeezed

1 Tbsp. chives, minced

Pinch of sea salt, to taste

1/2 cup wild rice, cooked according to package instructions

1 tsp. butter, divided

1/2 tsp. olive oil

1 cup raw shrimps, shelled, deveined, drained

Directions:

1. Pour 1/2 tsp. butter and oil into wok set over medium heat.
2. Add in shrimps and peas. Sauté until shrimps are coral pink, about 5 to 7 minutes.
3. Add in wild rice and cook until well heated through.
4. Season with salt and butter.
5. Transfer to a plate. Sprinkle chives and lemon juice on top. Serve.

Valencia Salad

Ingredients:

1 small satsuma or tangerine, pulp only

1 tsp. white wine vinegar

1 tsp. extra virgin olive oil

1 pinch fresh thyme, minced

Pinch of sea salt

Pinch of black pepper, to taste

1 tsp. Kalamata olives in oil, pitted, drained lightly, halved, julienned

1 head, small Romaine lettuce, rinsed, spun-dried, sliced into bite-sized pieces

1 piece, small shallot, julienned

1 tsp. Dijon mustard

Directions:

1. Combine vinegar, oil, fresh thyme, salt, mustard, black pepper, and honey, if using. Whisk well until dressing emulsifies a little.
2. Toss together remaining salad ingredients in a salad bowl.
3. Drizzle dressing on top when about to serve. Serve immediately with 1 slice if sugar-free sourdough bread or saltine.

Tenderloin Stir Fry With Red And Green Grapes

Ingredients:

1/2 cup green grapes, quartered

1/2 cup red grapes, quartered

black peppercorns, freshly cracked

1 tsp. apple cider vinegar, freshly juiced

1 medallion, 6 oz. pork tenderloin, trimmed well, remove membrane

sea salt sesame oil

For grape vinaigrette

Directions:

1. To make the vinaigrette, toss ingredients in a bowl. Chill prior to serving.
2. Meanwhile, preheat stovetop or electric grill for at least 3 minutes.
3. Lightly season pork with salt and sesame oil.
4. Grill only until well seared on both sides, about 10 to 12 minutes.
5. Remove from grill. Tent with aluminium foil, and allow the meat to rest 5 minutes.
6. Place cooked pork medallion on a plate. Top off with vinaigrette. Serve.

Aioli With Eggs

Ingredients:

1/2 cup lemon juice, fresh squeezed, pips removed

1/2 tsp. sea salt

Dash of cayenne pepper powder

Pinch of white pepper, to taste

2 fresh egg yolks

1 garlic, grated

2 Tbsp. water

1 cup extra virgin olive oil

Directions:

1. Pour garlic, fresh egg yolks, salt and water into blender; process until smooth.
2. Drizzle in olive oil in a slow stream until dressing emulsifies.
3. Add in remaining ingredients. Taste; adjust seasoning if needed.
4. Pour into an airtight container; use as needed.

Simple Yet Effective Vegan Truffle

1 a cup of cocoa nibs

1 a cup of agave nectar

2 teaspoons of vanilla extract

1 teaspoon of salt

1 and a 1/2 cups unsweetened coconut, shredded

2 cups of Mejdool dates

1 cup of raw almonds

2 and a 1/2 cups of raw cocoa powder

Directions:

1. Pre-heat your oven to 350-degree Fahrenheit
2. Spread out the coconut on a baking sheet

3. Line another baking sheet with parchment paper
4. Bake the coconut in your oven for about 10 minutes, making sure to keep stirring them from time to time
5. Take a food processor and add dates, almonds and process until smooth
6. Add cocoa powder and process until mixed well
7. Transfer mix to a bowl
8. Fold 1 cup of your toasted coconut, agave nectar, salt and vanilla extract into the date mix. Mix well
9. Roll up the dough into tablespoon sized balls and roll them in the remaining toasted truffle balls.
10. Transfer the balls to your parchment lined baking sheet and allow them to harden for about 60 minutes
11. Enjoy!

Guilt And Dairy "Free" Chocolate Pudding

Ingredients:

1/2 teaspoon of vanilla extract

1/2 cup of white sugar

1/2 cup of unsweetened cocoa powder

 3 tablespoons of cornstarch

2 tablespoons of water

1 and a 1 cups of soy milk

Directions:

1. Take a small sized bowl and add cornstarch and water and mix well to form a nice paste like texture

2. Take a large sized saucepan and place it over medium heat
3. Add soy milk, sugar, vanilla, cocoa and your prepared cornstarch mixture
4. Give the whole mixture a stir and allow it to cook until boiling point is reached
5. Keep stirring until the mixture is thick
6. Remove the heat Allow it to cool and chill in your fridge until it is fully cooled and has settled in Enjoy!

A Very Subtle Cherry Crisp

Ingredients:

¾ teaspoon cinnamon, ground

¾ teaspoon of nutmeg, ground

1/2 cup pecans, chopped

1/3 cup of melted margarine

4 ounce of cherry pie filling

1 a cup of all-purpose flour

1 a cup of rolled oats 1/2 cup of brown sugar

Directions:

1. Pre-heat your oven to 350-degree Fahrenheit
2. Take a 2-quart baking dish and carefully grease it up.
3. Pour the pie filling mixture evenly into the dish and spread it up Take a medium sized bowl and add flour, sugar, oats, cinnamon and nutmeg
4. Add melted margarine and mix, spread this mixture over your pie filling. Sprinkle chopped up pecans
5. Bake for 30 minutes until the top shows a golden-brown texture
6. Allow it to cool for about 15 minutes and enjoy!

Delicious Pumpkin Pie "Spicy" Pastries

Ingredients:

1 tablespoon of melted Vegan butter

2 tablespoons of packed brown sugar

1 and a 1 teaspoon of pumpkin pie spice

1 a pack of rolled up unbaked pie crust (Vegan Compliant)

How To

1. Pre-heat you oven to a temperature of 450 degree Fahrenheit
2. Unroll the pie crust according to the package direction following the microwave method.
3. Place it on a lightly flour surface

4. Brush up the pie crust with melted butter
5. Sprinkle with pie spice and brown sugar
6. Take a pizza cutter and cut up the dough into 1 inch squares.
7. Take an ungreased large cookie sheet and transfer them to the sheet, making sure to leave some space between the pieces.
8. Bake for about 8 minutes until they are golden brown. Serve and enjoy!

Cool And Warm Oven Roasted Plums

Ingredients:

1 a teaspoon of cinnamon, ground

1/8 teaspoon of nutmeg, ground

1/8 teaspoon of cumin

1/8 teaspoon of cardamom

1/2 cup of toasted and slivered almonds

Cook Directions

1 a cup of orange juice

4 pieces of plums, pitted and halved

2 tablespoons of packed brown sugar

Pre-heat your oven to 400-degree Fahrenheit

1. Take a shallow baking dish and grease it with Cook spray. Add your

plums to the pan with the cut side facing up

2. Take a bowl and whisk in orange juice, cinnamon, brown sugar, cumin, nutmeg and cardamom.

3. Drizzle the mixture over your plums. Bake for 25 minutes until the plums are hot and the sauce shows a bubbly texture

4. Top with some almonds and enjoy!

Apples With A Fire Within

Ingredients:

Cored granny smith apple

1 tablespoon of brown sugar

1/2 teaspoon of ground cinnamon

Cook Directions

Core the apples well and fill them up with cinnamon and brown sugar

Wrap the apples using a large piece of heavy foil(making sure to make a few extra twist to make a handle)

Place the apples in a coal of campfire (or BBQ) and allow them to cook for about 5-10 minutes

Gently unwrap the apples and serve!

Awesome And Crunchy Muffins

Ingredients:

2 cups of coconut, unsweetened, shredded

1 teaspoon of salt

1 tablespoon of white sugar

2 and a 1 cups of coconut milk

1 tablespoon of water

1 and a 1/2 cup of white rice flour

Directions

1. Pre-heat your oven to 375 degree Fahrenheit

2. Take mini muffin tins and spray with Cook spray
3. Take a bowl and add coconut milk and water
4. Stir in white rice flour, salt and shredded coconut
5. Spoon up the mixture into your prepped mini muffin cups and sprinkle sugar on top
6. Bake in your pre-heated oven for 30 minutes until the tops are golden brown

The Cherry Beet Delight

Ingredients

1 cup water, filtered, alkaline

1 cup coconut milk

Pinch of organic vanilla powder

Pinch of cinnamon

Pinch of stevia

1 cup cherries, pitted

1 cup beets Few fresh Banana slices

Few mint leaves/lime slices to garnish h

Directions:

1. Add berries, beets, water, fresh Banana slices, coconut milk to your blender
2. Blend well until smooth

3. Add more water if the texture is too creamy for you
4. Add coconut oil, vanilla, cinnamon and stir
5. Add a bit of stevia for extra sweetness
6. Garnish with mint leaves and lime slices
7. Enjoy!

Green Delight

Ingredients:

1 tablespoon MCT oil

1 tablespoon chia seeds

1 and 1 cups water

¾ cup whole almond milk yogurt

2 cups 5 – lettuce mix salad greens

1 pack stevia

Directions:

1. Add listed Ingredients to blender
2. Blend until you have a smooth and creamy texture
3. Serve chilled and enjoy!

Easy Chia Seed Pumpkin Pudding

Ingredients

1 cup pumpkin puree

1 and 1/2 cup almond milk

1 cup chia seeds

1 cup pure maple syrup

2 teaspoons pumpkin spice

Directions:

1. Add all of the ingredients to a bowl and gently stir
2. Let it refrigerate overnight or for at least 15 minutes
3. Top with your desired ingredients such as blueberries, almonds, etc.
4. Serve and enjoy!

The Mediterranean Fruit Granita

Ingredients

1/2 cup orange juice 2 tablespoons lemon juice

1 cup raspberries 1 cup brown sugar

2 pound ripe nectarines

Directions

1. Take a pan and a place it over medium-high heat
2. Add water and sugar, add the fruits and bring to a boil.
3. Boil everything for 10 minutes. Stir in raspberries.
4. Add juice and extra sugar if needed.

5. Remove the heat and transfer the mixture to your fridge, let it chill for 30 minutes
6. Serve and enjoy!

Guilt Free Lemon And Rosemary Drink

Ingredients:

1 tablespoon lemon juice, fresh

1 tablespoon pepitas

1 tablespoon flaxseed, ground

1 and 1 cups water

1 cup whole almond milk yogurt

1 cup Garden greens

1 pack stevia

1 tablespoon olive oil

1 stalk fresh rosemary

Directions:

1. Add listed Ingredients to blender
2. Blend until you have a smooth and creamy texture
3. Serve chilled and enjoy!

Strawberry And Rhubarb Smoothie

Ingredients:

1 cup plain Greek strawberries

Pinch of ground cinnamon

3 ice cubes

1 rhubarb stalk, chopped

1 cup fresh strawberries, sliced

Directions:

1. Take a small saucepan and fill with water over high heat
2. Bring to boil and add rhubarb, boil for 3 minutes
3. Drain and transfer to a blender
4. Add strawberries, honey, yogurt, cinnamon and pulse mixture until smooth

5. Add ice cubes and blend until thick and has no lumps
6. Pour into glass and enjoy chilled

Vanilla Hemp Drink

Ingredients:

1 cup frozen blueberries, mixed

4 cup leafy greens, kale and spinach

1 tablespoons flaxseed

1 tablespoon almond butter

1 cup water

1 cup unsweetened hemp almond milk, vanilla

1 and 1 tablespoons coconut oil, unrefined

Directions:

1. Add listed Ingredients to blender
2. Blend until you have a smooth and creamy texture
3. Serve chilled and enjoy!

Yogurt And Kale Smoothie

Ingredients:

1 tablespoon MCT oil

1 tablespoon sunflower seed

1 cup water

1 cup whole almond milk yogurt

1 cup baby kale greens

1 pack stevia

Directions:

1. Add listed Ingredients to blender
2. Blend until you have a smooth and creamy texture
3. Serve chilled and enjoy!

Spiced Kale Chips

Ingredients:

1/8 tsp. Black Pepper

1/2 tsp. Cayenne Pepper, grounded

1 tsp. Oil

1 Bunch of Kale, washed & patted dry

1/8 tsp. Garlic Powder

1/2 tsp. Salt

Directions:

1. Preheat the oven to 300 ° F.
2. After that, tear off the kale leaves and place them on a wire rack, which is on top of a foil-lined baking sheet.
3. Now, apply oil in your hands and massage them on the leaves.
4. Tip: You need to use the oil only lightly.
5. Top it with salt, pepper, and cayenne pepper.
6. Finally, bake them for 25 minutes or until the edges are crispy.
7. Tip: If you wish it to be spicier, you can add more cayenne pepper.

Vegetable Nuggets

Ingredients:

2 cups Broccoli Florets 1 cup Almond Meal

1 cup Carrots, chopped coarsely 1/2 tsp. Salt

1 tsp. Garlic, minced

1 tsp. Turmeric, grounded

1/2 tsp. Black Pepper

2 cups Cauliflower Florets

1 Egg, large & pastured

Directions:

1. To make these tasty nuggets, you first need to preheat the oven to 450 ° F. Next, place broccoli, turmeric,

cauliflower, black pepper, carrots, sea salt, and turmeric in a food processor.

2. Pulse them for a minute or until you get a finely grounded mixture.

3. Then, stir in the almond meal and fresh egg into it and pulse them again until mixed.

4. Now, transfer the veggie-almond mixture to a large mixing bowl.

5. Scoop out the mixture with a tablespoon and make circular discs with your hands.

6. After that, place the discs on the parchment paper-lined baking sheet.

7. Finally, bake them for 25 to 25 minutes while flipping it once.

Cabbage Pineapple Slaw

Ingredients:

For the sauce: 1 cup Cashews, soaked

1 tsp. Red Pepper Flakes

1 cup Water 2-inches Ginger

1 tbsp. + 1 tsp. Lime Juice

Salt & Pepper, to taste

2 Red Bell Peppers, sliced thinly

1 of 1 Purple Cabbage, thinly sliced

1 cup Cilantro, sliced thinly

1 of 1 Red Cabbage, sliced thinly

3 cups Pineapple, chopped

Directions:

1. To begin with, place all the ingredients needed to make the sauce in a high-speed blender until you get a smooth sauce.
2. After that, place both the cabbage slices, pineapple, and red peppers in a large mixing bowl. Toss well.
3. To this, spoon in the cashew sauce and toss them again.
4. Serve immediately or keep in refrigerator until served.
5. Tip: You can even add tuna or chicken to this salad for a main dish.

Turmeric Muffins

Ingredients:

1/3 cup Maple Syrup

1 tsp. Baking Soda

1 tsp. Vanilla Extract

2 tsp. Turmeric

¾ cup + 2 tbsp. Coconut Flour

6 Eggs, large & preferably pastured

1 tsp. Ginger Powder

1 cup Coconut Milk, unsweetened

Dash of Salt & Pepper

Directions:

1. Preheat the oven to 350 ° F.
2. After that, mix eggs, vanilla extract, milk, maple syrup, and milk in a large mixing bowl until combined well.
3. In another bowl, combine turmeric, coconut flour, ginger powder, baking soda, pepper, and salt.
4. Now, stir in the coconut flour mixture gradually to the milk mixture until you get a smooth batter.
5. Then, pour the smooth mixture to paper-lined muffin pan while distributing it evenly.
6. Finally, bake them for 25 to 25 minutes or until slightly browned at the edges.
7. Allow the muffins to cool completely.
8. Tip: They are freezer friendly and stay good for one month.

Coffee Protein Bars

Ingredients:

18 Medjool Dates, large & pitted

1/2 cup Cocoa Powder, unsweetened

3 tbsp. Instant Coffee

2 cups Nuts 5 tbsp. Water

1 cup Fresh egg White Protein Powder

Directions:

1. First, blend nuts, instant coffee, fresh egg white protein powder, and cocoa in a food processor until broken down into smaller pieces.
2. After that, stir in the dates and process them again.
3. Then, spoon in one tablespoon of water gradually to the processor

while it is running or until you get a sticky mixture.

4. Now, transfer the mixture to a parchment paper-lined baking sheet and spread it across evenly.

5. Next, place the baking sheet in the refrigerator for 2 1 ½ hour or until set. Slice them into bars. Tip: If you prefer, you can add cacao nibs.

Cauliflower Popcorn

Ingredients:

Salt, as needed

2 tsp. Extra Virgin Olive Oil

4 cups Cauliflower, broken into florets

Directions:

1. First, toss together the cauliflower florets and extra virgin olive oil in a large mixing bowl until coated well.
2. To this, spoon in the salt and toss well.
3. Next, bake them for 28 to 30 minutes at 450 ° F or until browned and tender.
4. Serve with more extra olive oil if needed.

Spiced Pumpkin Seeds

Ingredients:

1 tsp. Celtic Sea Salt 2 tsp. Olive Oil

1 tbsp. Chili Powder

1 cup Pumpkin Seeds

Directions:

1. To start with, keep the pumpkin seeds in a large-sized iron cast skillet over medium-high heat.
2. Roast them for 3 minutes while stirring it frequently.
3. After that, take the skillet from the heat and to this, spoon in the chili powder and sea salt.
4. Toss well.

5. Finally, allow it to cool completely and serve.

Curry Roasted Chickpeas

Ingredients:

15 oz. Garbanzo Beans or Chickpeas, washed & drained

1 tsp. Sea Salt

1 tbsp. Olive Oil

2 tsp. Curry Powder

Directions:

1. First, preheat the oven to 450 ° F.
2. Next, place the chickpeas, salt, olive oil, and curry powder in a large mixing bowl and combine them well.
3. Now, transfer the seasoned chickpeas to a baking sheet and spread them in a single layer.
4. After that, bake them for 25 to 30 minutes or until crispy while turning them once in between.
5. Allow them to cool completely and serve.

Coconut Oats Balls

Ingredients:

15 cup Coconut Flakes, unsweetened

1 cup Almonds, chopped

1 cup Peanut Butter

1/2 cup Honey

2 cups Steel Oats 2 tsp. Vanilla Extract

Directions:

1. For making these energy balls, you first need to place the oats in the food processor and then process them until broken down.
2. Next, combine the rest of the ingredients in a large mixing bowl until everything comes together.

3. Now, by using your hands, make balls out of this smooth dough. Then, place the balls in the refrigerator for half an hour or until set.

Seasoned Coconut Flakes

Ingredients:

1 tsp. Coconut Oil 1/2 tsp. Allspice

1 tsp. Cinnamon 1/2 tsp. Salt

1/2 tsp. Nutmeg

1 cup Coconut Flakes, unsweetened

Directions:

1. Preheat the oven to 350 ° F.
2. After that, place all the ingredients needed to make the savory snacks, excluding the coconut oil in a large zip lock bags. Shake well. Next, spoon in the coconut oil to the bag and shake again, so the seasoning coats the coconut flakes.

3. Now, transfer the seasoned coconut to a greased baking sheet.
4. Then, place the sheet in the middle rack and bake the coconut flakes for 4 to 5 minutes. Tip: Make sure not to over bake them.
5. Finally, remove the sheet from the oven immediately and allow it to cool completely before serving.

Turmeric Bars

Ingredients:

12 teaspoon turmeric powder

2 teaspoons honey

1/8 teaspoon black pepper

1 cup shredded coconut

10 dates, pitted 1 tablespoon coconut oil

1 teaspoon cinnamon 10 cup coconut butter

Directions:

1. Prepare a baking pan a nd line with parchment paper.
2. Place the cocon ut and dates in a food processor and pulse unti l well-combined.
3. Add in the coconut oil and cinnamon.

4. Press the dough at the bottom of the pan and allow to set in the fridge for 2 hours.
5. Make the filling by melting the coconut butter in a double boiler. Stir in turmeric powder and honey. Pour in the mixtu reinto the pan with the crust.
6. Allow to set in the fridge for at least 2 hours.

Anti-Inflammatory Turmeric Gummies

Ingredients:

8 tablespoons unflavored gelatin powder

3 1 cups water

1 teaspoon ground turmeric

6 tablespoons maple syrup

Directions:

1. In a pot, combine the water, turmeric, and maple syrup.
2. Bring to a boil for 5 minutes.
3. Remove from the heat and sprinkle with gelatin powder.
4. Mix to hydrate the gelatin.
5. Turn on the heat and bring to a boil until the gelatin is completely dissolved.

6. Pour the mixture in a dish and chill the mixture in the fridge for at least 4 hours.
7. Once set, slice into small squares.

Ginger Spiced Mixed Nuts

Ingredients:

pumpkin seeds, cashew, etc.)

1 teaspoon grated ginger

1 teaspoon salt

2 large fresh egg whites, pasture-raised

2 cups mixed nuts (raw almond,

Directions:

1. Preheat the oven to 2500F.
2. Whip the fresh egg whites until frothy. Add in ginger and salt.
3. Add in the mixed nuts into the fresh egg mixture. Stir to coat everything.
4. Place parchment paper in a baking tray and spread the nuts evenly on to the sheet.

5. Bake for 45 minutes.
6. Allow the mixture to cool and harden.
7. Break into pieces and store in the fridge until ready to consume

Spicy Tuna Rolls

Ingredients:

2 slices avocado, diced

1/8 teaspoon salt

1/8 teaspoon pepper

1 medium cucumber

1 can yellowfin tuna, wild-caught

Directions:

1. Use a mandolin to thinly slice the cucumber lengthwise.
2. In a mixing bowl, combine the tuna and avocado. Season with salt and pepper to taste.

3. Spoon the tuna and avocado mixture and spread evenly on cucumber slices.
4. Roll the cucumber slices and secure the ends with toothpicks.
5. Allow to chill in the fridge before serving.

Veggie Burrito

Ingredients:

1/3 cup red onions, sliced thinly

1/2 cup avocado meat

1 cup cooked quinoa 1/2 teaspoon salt

1/2 cup cilantro leaves, chopped

1 teaspoon avocado oil

4 medium collard greens, stalks trimmed

1/3 cup bell pepper, julienned

1/3 cup chopped tomatoes

Directions:

1. Bring water to a boil and blanch the collard greens.
2. Set aside. In a skillet, heat the avocado oil over medium flame and sauté the bell pepper for 1 minute. Set aside.
3. Assemble the burrito by placing the blanched collard greens on a flat surface.
4. Place the bell pepper, tomatoes, onions, avocado meat, and quinoa in the center. Add in the cilantro leaves.
5. Roll the collard greens to create a burrito.

Nutrition:

Calories 175 Cal Carbs 25 g

Protein 5 g Fiber: 5 g

Tasty Turkey Baked Balls

Ingredients:

2 Tbsp parsley, freshly chopped

3-Tbsps milk or water

A dash of salt and pepper

A pinch of freshly grated nutmeg

2 pound ground turkey

1 cup fresh breadcrumbs, white or whole wheat

1 cup Parmesan cheese, freshly grated

1 Tbsp basil, freshly chopped

1 Tbsp oregano, freshly chopped

2 pc large egg, beaten

Directions:

1. Preheat your oven to 350°F. Line two baking pans with parchment paper.
2. Stir in all of the ingredients in a large mixing bowl.
3. Form 2 inch balls from the mixture and place each ball in the baking pan.
4. Put the pan in the oven.
5. Bake for 30 minutes, or until the turkey cooks through and the surfaces turn brown.
6. Turn the meatballs once halfway into the cooking.

Chicken, Corn & Spinach Sauté

Ingredients:

2 pc zucchini, cubed 2 tsp cumin

2-cups baby spinach leaves

Juice of one lime 1/2 cup goat cheese, crumbled

Salt and pepper, to taste

2 Tbsp olive oil

2 clove garlic, minced

2-pc chicken breasts, sliced 1 cup corn kernels

Directions:

1. Sauté the chicken with garlic and olive oil in a skillet placed over medium high heat Cook for about a minute until the chicken turns brown. Remove the chicken from the pan.
2. Set aside. In the same skillet, add in the corn and zucchini, and cook for a minute until the zucchini is tender.
3. Add the cumin, and stir while cooking further for one more minute.
4. Put the browned chicken back into the skillet, and cook until done.
5. Stir in the lime juice and spinach, and keep cooking until the spinach wilts.
6. Sprinkle with salt and pepper.
7. Just before serving, stir in the goat cheese.

Sprouts & Slices In Wheat Wrap

Ingredients:

⅛-cup red onions, diced

1/2 cup mozzarella, partly skimmed, shredded

1/2 cup hummus or guacamole dressing

2 pc whole-wheat wrap, large

1/2 cup carrots, grated

1 cup romaine lettuce, shredded

1 pc cucumber, sliced round, then halved

1 cup bean sprouts 1/2 cup tomatoes, diced

Directions:

1. In a medium-sized mixing bowl, prepare the dressing or spread by combining all of the ingredients excluding the cheese and wrap.
2. Mix well until thoroughly combined.
3. On a clean table, spread out the whole-wheat wrap.
4. Spread the dressing evenly on the wrap. Be sure to leave a couple of inches on one end of the wrap for folding.
5. Add the cheese to an even layer over the spread. Fold over the full wrap and tuck in at the bottom.

Feta-Filled & Tomato-Topped Turkey Burger Bites

Ingredients:

1 cup tomatoes, sun-dried, diced

1 cup Feta cheese, low fat

2-Tbsps green onions or chives, diced

2 lb turkey, lean, ground

1 tsp black pepper

Kosher or sea salt to taste

Directions:

1. Stir in all the listed ingredients in a mixing bowl.
2. Mix well until blended thoroughly.

137

3. Divide the mixture evenly into four patties. Store them in the refrigerator.
4. When cooking time comes, you can either grill or fry the frozen patties for about 10 minutes each on both sides.
5. Serve by topping the burgers with your preferred condiments.

Simply Sautéed Flaky Fillet

Ingredients:

2 pc lemon, juice

Salt and pepper to taste

1/2 cup parsley or cilantro, chopped

6-fillets tilapia

2-Tbsps olive oil

Directions:

1. Sauté tilapia fillets with olive oil in a medium-sized skillet placed over medium heat.
2. Cook for 4 minutes on each side until the fish flakes easily with a fork.
3. Add salt and pepper to taste. Pour the lemon juice to each fillet.

4. To serve, sprinkle the cooked fillets with chopped parsley or cilantro.

Spicy Sautéed Chinese Chicken

Ingredients:

For the Marinade:

2 Tbsp garlic-chili sauce or chili paste

2 Tbsp Hoisin sauce 2 Tbsp light soy sauce

2 Tbsp ginger, peeled and minced

For the Chicken:

11 Tbsps canola oil

2 lb chicken breasts, boneless, skinless, cubed

Directions:

1. Whisk all the marinade ingredients altogether in a mixing bowl.
2. Add in the chicken pieces, and toss lightly to coat the chicken uniformly with the marinade.
3. Cover the bowl. Chill in the refrigerator for 25 minutes.
4. Sauté the chicken pieces with canola oil in a medium-sized pan placed over medium high heat.
5. Cook for about 5 minutes until its juices run clear and cook through.
6. To serve, place the cooked chicken over a choice of either cooked quinoa or brown rice noodles, or brown rice.

Tasty Thai Chicken In Crisp Cups

Ingredients:

- 2 Tbsp fish sauce 1 pc lime, juiced
- 2 tsp soy sauce, reduced-sodium
- 2 head iceberg lettuce, separated into cups
- A handful of cilantro and mint, finely chopped
- 11 Tbsps cooking oil
- 1 lb chicken breast, ground 2-pcs shallots, diced 1/2 pc red onion, diced 2 clove garlic, finely minced
- Jalapeño or Fresno chilies, freshly minced

Directions:

1. Sauté the ground chicken with a tablespoon of olive oil in a large wok placed over high heat.
2. Cook for about 3 minutes until the surfaces of the ground chicken turn brown.
3. Push the browned ground chicken to one side of the wok, and pour in the remaining oil.
4. Add in the shallots, red onion, garlic, and fresh chilies.
5. Sauté these added ingredients for about half a minute until effusing their fragrance.
6. Pour in the sauce, juice of one lime, and soy sauce.
7. Stir the entire mixture, including the ground chicken until cooked thoroughly.

8. To serve, distribute the cooked mixture evenly in lettuce cups.

Zesty Zucchini & Chicken In Classic Santa Fe Stir-Fry

Ingredients:

1 cup carrots, shredded

2 tsp paprika, smoked 2 tsp cumin, ground

1 tsp chili powder 1/2 tsp sea salt

2-Tbsp fresh lime juice

1/2 cup cilantro, freshly chopped

Brown rice or quinoa, when serving

2 Tbsp olive oil

2-pcs chicken breasts, sliced

2 pc onion, small, diced

2-cloves garlic, minced 2 pc zucchini, diced

Directions:

1. Sauté the chicken with olive oil for about 3 minutes until the chicken turns brown.
2. Set aside. Use the same wok and add the fresh onion and garlic.
3. Cook until the fresh onion is tender. Add in the carrots and zucchini. Stir the mixture, and cook further for about a minute.
4. Add all the seasonings into the mix, and stir to cook for another minute.
5. Return the chicken in the wok, and pour in the lime juice.
6. Stir to cook until everything cooks through.
7. To serve, place the mixture over cooked rice or quinoa and top with the freshly chopped cilantro.

Crispy Cheese-Crusted Fish Fillet

Ingredients:

1/2 tsp sea salt

1/2 tsp ground pepper

2 Tbsp olive oil

4-pcs tilapia fillets

1/2 cup whole-wheat breadcrumbs

1/2 cup Parmesan cheese, grated

Directions:

1. Preheat the oven to 375°F.
2. Stir in the breadcrumbs, Parmesan cheese, salt, pepper, and olive oil in a mixing bowl. Mix well until blended thoroughly.
3. Coat the fillets with the mixture, and lay each on a lightly sprayed baking

147

sheet. Place the sheet in the oven. Bake for 10 minutes until the fillets cook through and turn brownish.

Sautéed Shrimp Jambalaya Jumble

Ingredients:

1 tsp Worcestershire sauce

⅔-cup carrots, chopped

11/2 cups chicken sausage, precooked and diced

2-cups lentils, soaked overnight and precooked

2-cups okra, chopped

A dash of crushed red pepper and black pepper

10-oz. medium shrimp, peeled

1/2 cup celery, chopped 1 cup onion, chopped

2 Tbsp oil or butter 1/2 tsp garlic, minced

1/2 tsp fresh onion salt or sea salt

⅓-cup tomato sauce 1 tsp smoked paprika

Directions:

1. Sauté the shrimp, celery, and fresh onion with oil in a pan placed over medium high heat for five minutes, or until the shrimp turn pinkish.
2. Add in the rest of the ingredients, and sauté further for 10 minutes, or until the veggies are tender.
3. To serve, divide the jambalaya mixture equally among four serving bowls. Top with pepper and cheese, if desired.

Toasted Tilapia Topped With Panko & Pecans

Ingredients:

2-tsps chopped fresh rosemary

A pinch of cayenne pepper

2 unit fresh egg white 4 x 4-oz. tilapia fillets

⅛-tsp salt

⅓-cup pecans, chopped

⅓-cup whole-wheat panko breadcrumbs

1 tsp coconut palm sugar 11 tsps olive oil

Directions:

1. Preheat your oven to 350°F. Stir in the first seven ingredients in a small baking dish.
2. Mix well until thoroughly combined.
3. Put the dish in the oven. Bake for 8 minutes or until the mixture turns brown.
4. Set aside. Increase the heat to 400°F. Meanwhile, grease a large baking dish with cooking spray.
5. Whisk the fresh egg white in a shallow bowl.
6. Dip the fillet, one at a time, in the bowl of whisked egg.
7. Dredge the soaked fillet in the pecan mixture, coating each side lightly. Place each coated fillet in the large baking dish.
8. Put the dish in the oven, and bake for 10 minutes, or until the fillets cook through.

Tortilla Tostadas With Peppered Potato & Kingly Kale

Ingredients:

12-pcs Brussels sprouts, finely chopped

2 tsp honey

2 Tbsp lime juice

Corn tortillas

A drizzle of yogurt

2-pcs medium sweet potatoes, cleaned and chopped

A pinch of cayenne pepper

3-Tbsps olive oil (divided)

8-stems kale, roughly chopped

A pinch of salt

Directions:

1. Preheat your oven to 400°F. Line two baking sheets with aluminum foil.
2. Toss the sweet potatoes with cayenne pepper and 2-tablespoons of oil on the first baking sheet.
3. In the other baking sheet, toss the kale with salt and oil.
4. Put both sheets in the oven. Roast the potatoes for 45 minutes. Roast the kale for 10 minutes until, or until the edges turn crispy, but not browned.
5. Meanwhile, toss the sprouts with the honey and lime juice.
6. Set aside.
7. Place the corn tortillas on a piece of tin foil, and toast in the warm oven for 3 minutes.
8. To serve, scoop equally the sweet potatoes and crispy kale among four tortillas. Top each tortilla with the

sprout's slaw. Drizzle with yogurt, mint, and toasted coconut, if desired.

Turkey Tomato Sweet Potato Stuffed Peppers

Ingredients:

1 cup homemade tomato sauce

Crushed red pepper flakes (optional)

A dash of salt and pepper

2-pcs big bell peppers, sliced in half

2 tbsp extra-virgin olive oil

2-cups ground turkey, grass-fed

2-cloves garlic, minced

1 cup onions, diced

1⅔-cups sweet potato, diced

Directions:

1. Preheat your oven to 350°F. Meanwhile, grease a baking dish with cooking spray.
2. Heat the oil in a skillet placed over medium high heat. Sauté the garlic and turkey for 10 minutes or until the meat is no longer pink, stirring occasionally.
3. Add the onions, and cook further for 3 minutes, or until the onions turn golden brown.
4. Add the sweet potato, and cover the skillet.
5. Cook the potatoes for 8 minutes, or until they are tender.
6. Pour the tomato sauce, pepper flakes, and a dash of salt and pepper to taste. Set aside.
7. Arrange the halved bell peppers in the baking dish, with their cavity

sides facing up. Stuff each half with the cooked mixture.

8. Put the dish in the oven. Roast for half an hour until the bell peppers become tender.

Baked Buffalo Cauliflower Chunks

Ingredients:

2 pc medium cauliflower, cut into bite-size pieces

1 cup hot sauce

2-Tbsps butter, melted

1/2 cup water

1/2 cup fresh Banana flour

A pinch of salt and pepper

Directions:

1. Preheat your oven to 425°F. Meanwhile, line a baking pan with foil.
2. Combine the water, flour, and a pinch of salt and pepper in a large mixing

bowl. Mix well until thoroughly combined.

3. Add the cauliflower; toss to coat thoroughly. Transfer the mixture to the baking pan. Bake for 15 minutes, flipping once.

4. While baking, combine the hot sauce and butter in a small bowl. Pour the sauce over the baked cauliflower.

5. Return the baked cauliflower to the oven, and bake further for 25 minutes. Serve immediately with a ranch dressing on the side, if desired.

Cool Garbanzo And Spinach Beans

Ingredients

1 tablespoon olive oil

1 onion, diced

10 ounces spinach, chopped

12 ounces garbanzo beans

Take a skillet and add olive oil, let it warm over medium-low heat

Add onions, garbanzo and cook for 5 minutes

Stir in spinach, cumin, garbanzo beans and season with salt

Use a spoon to smash gently

Cook thoroughly until heated, enjoy!

1 teaspoon cumin

Lemony Garlic Shrimp

Ingredients

1/2 cup lemon juice

2 tablespoons olive oil

1/2 cup parsley

1 and 1/2 pounds shrimp, boiled or steamed

3 tablespoons garlic, minced

Directions:

1. Take a small skillet and place it over medium heat, add garlic and oil and stir cook for 1 minute

2. Add parsley, lemon juice and season with salt and pepper accordingly
3. Add shrimp in a large bowl and transfer the mixture from the skillet over the shrimp
4. Chill and serve

Coconut And Hazelnut Chilled Glass

Ingredients:

1 and 1 cups water

1 pack stevia

1 cup coconut almond milk

1/2 cup hazelnuts, chopped

Directions

1. Add listed Ingredients to blender
2. Blend until you have a smooth and creamy texture
3. Serve chilled and enjoy!

Coriander Greens With Zucchini Sauté!

Ingredients

3 garlic cloves, minced

2 tablespoons tamari sauce

4 tablespoons avocado oil

10 ounces beef, sliced into 2 2-inch strips

1 zucchini, cut into 2-inch strips

1/2 cup parsley, chopped

Directions:

1. Add 2 tablespoons avocado oil in a frying pan over high heat

2. Place strips of beef and brown for a few minutes on high heat
3. Once the meat is brown, add zucchini strips and Saute until tender
4. Once tender, add tamari sauce, garlic, parsley and let them sit for a few minutes more
5. Serve immediately and enjoy!

Walnuts And Asparagus Delight

Ingredients

1 and 1 tablespoons olive oil

¾ pound asparagus, trimmed

1/2 cup walnuts, chopped

Sunflower seeds and pepper to taste

Directions

1. Place a skillet over medium heat add olive oil and let it heat up
2. Add asparagus, Sauté for 10 minutes until browned
3. Season with sunflower seeds and pepper

4. Remove heat
5. Add walnuts and toss
6. Serve warm!

Butternut Squash With Lentils

Ingredients

 Coconut milk – 1 (13.5 ounce) can

Vegetable broth –15 to 2 cups

Lentils – 1 (15-ounce) can lentils, drained and rinsed

Chopped fresh parsley – 1/2 cup

Chopped fresh sage – 2 Tbsps.

Chopped toasted walnuts - 1 cup

Coconut oil – 1 Tbsp.

Fresh onion – 1, chopped Garlic – 2 cloves, minced

Small butternut squash – 1, cut into 1 inch cubes

Packed spinach – 4 cups Salt – 1 tsp.

Ground black pepper – 1 tsp.

Directions:

1. Preheat the oven to 375F.
2. Melt the coconut oil in a skillet. Add the garlic and onion.
3. Sauté for 3 minutes.
4. Add the spinach, butternut squash, salt, and pepper.
5. Sauté for 3 minutes more.
6. Stir in the coconut milk and just enough vegetable broth to cover the squash.
7. Bring the liquid to a boil.

8. Add the sage, parsley, and lentils. Stir to combine.
9. Place the skillet in the preheated oven and bake the casserole for 25 to 30 minutes, until the squash is tender.
10. Transfer the casserole to a serving dish and garnish with the walnuts.